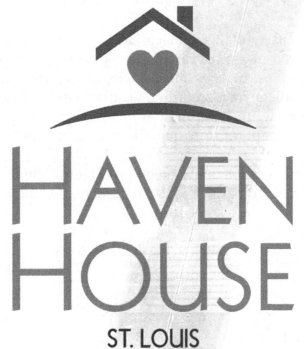

HAVEN HOUSE

ST. LOUIS

THE FIRST TWENTY YEARS

First edition published by Enigma Books, an imprint of Prince and Pauper Press, Clinton, MI.

ISBN: 978-1-62251-057-3

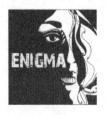

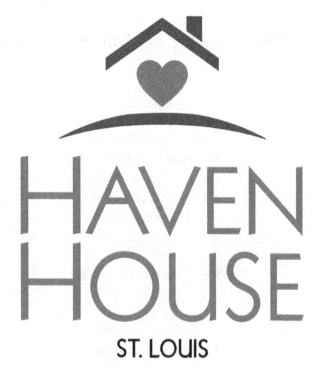

HAVEN HOUSE

ST. LOUIS

THE FIRST TWENTY YEARS

By Glenn Sartori

Other Books by Glenn Sartori

<u>Novels</u>
Epiphany
Union of Friends
Consequences of Falling
The Triplets' Secret
Her Father's Past
The Viewing

<u>Non-fiction</u>
First Jobs Remembered

<u>Memoirs</u>
Life on Alaska
Life on South Grand
Life on West Pine
Never Knew I Was a Dinosaur

Dedication

"To the families, staff and volunteers of HavenHouse St. Louis—past, present and future."

Epigraph

"As one person, I cannot change the world, but I can change the world of one person."

-Paul Shane Spear, Make-A-Wish Foundation

Table of Contents

First Foreword

I have had the pleasure and honor of working with Glenn Sartori dating back to the early 1990s, when he and Rosanne volunteered at the children's home. A few years later, he was appointed to the children's home board where I served as executive director. When the children's home stopped serving children directly, Glenn spearheaded the start of HavenHouse St. Louis (January 2005) and has continuously served on the board. As executive director of what was then a new non-profit and mission, I had much to learn. His passion, enthusiasm, and outstanding organizational skills were tremendous assets as board president. His passion and conviction, patience, sense of humor and writing and math acumen (his engineering background) mentored me and the staff to become skilled in our own rights.

Most of Glenn's writings and books have been reflections of his experiences. Collecting the twenty-year history of HavenHouse is a treasure I shall always value. In my many years as executive director, none was more rewarding than serving the families at HavenHouse and having the privilege of working with a dedicated board and staff who worked tirelessly to support the patients and families staying at HavenHouse, many of whom are still connected to the mission.

Who could have predicted the success and impact that HavenHouse has today? I'm looking forward to the next twenty years.

Kathy Sindel

Second Foreword

As we enter 2025, I will be entering my 17th year with HavenHouse St. Louis. Time has quickly passed, and the importance of our mission has only proven to be more needed and critically important to patients, families and caregivers who face traveling for their medical care and life-saving treatments. For many years, I served in an operational role for our organization. I've had many titles along the way! I'll test my memory here and see how this lands. In 2008, I was hired as the Director of Family Services and then moved to Program Director and as we enter our 20th year as an organization, I am proud and honored to lead a wonderful team and fulfill our mission as the Executive Director. It's fair to say that I was taught by the best, our former Executive Director and founder, Kathy Sindel. I worked alongside her for many years and feel so very lucky to have had that opportunity.

Working alongside Kathy meant working alongside Glenn and his wife, Rosanne. Within my first week, it was clear that Glenn was a steadfast, committed, empathetic, dedicated board member and supporter of HavenHouse. It was wonderful to see his commitment and his drive to help those we serve. Glenn and I share a funny story and that is of our water main break. I always go back to this day, and while I'll let Glenn do most of the sharing in the book, it's important to know that, neither one of us knew what to do! We were without water in the house. We had a house full of patients and families and unfortunately, we had to evacuate. Glenn came right over when he received my distress call. I'm sure it sounded like distress! We talked about a few options and his response is what sticks with me to this day. Glenn's response in the heat of the moment was, "How can I help? What do we need to do? I'll help in ANY way I can." That was exactly what I needed that day. He was there for me and while there wasn't anything anyone could do, Glenn was present, helpful (as he always is) and ready to jump in to help "in any way." Glenn is a treasured board member and has been a wonderful support system to me over the years. Especially, as a new Executive Director, navigating many unknowns, he has been consistently present. Glenn has received many calls from me in these last five years! Believe it or not, he still takes my call! We navigated Covid together and closing the house for eight weeks! We made it through and came out better in the end. I'm proud of that.

When Glenn shared the idea of writing a book about HavenHouse St. Louis I was thrilled. We have such a special mission. I couldn't think of a better way or a better person to share our milestones and history as we enter our 20th year and as we move into our new facility. It's a very exciting time for us as an organization and a perfect time to reflect and document our important history.

Hats off to you Glenn! Cheers to twenty years and twenty more! You have helped shape our leadership team from the beginning, and we wouldn't be celebrating all of these milestones if it weren't for you.

Paula Lowery

Introduction

The twentieth anniversary of HavenHouse is cause for celebration. It marks the opening of its new home and its stunning growth. The days when the St. Louis community asked, "What is HavenHouse?" are in the past. Instead, it is now a recognized, well-respected, valued premier hospital guest house.

This book tells the history of HavenHouse—its evolution from a nineteenth-century orphanage to a present-day home for families, who are on a stressful medical journey. There are many milestones and dates that mark key events in its growth, but more importantly, this book relates the warm, special story of the impact this organization has had on the St. Louis community and the families it continues to serve.

The heart of HavenHouse is certainly its mission—to provide the comfort of home and a community of support to patients and their families, who travel to St. Louis for medical care. But in order to fulfill that mission, it takes a caring staff, loads of volunteers, a dedicated board of directors, and the financial support of the community. The mission has been carried out at three locations—a building in West St. Louis County on Olive Boulevard, hotels in the

Westport area, and now, a building in midtown St. Louis on Park Avenue.

In January 2005, the State of Missouri awarded HavenHouse its 501(c)(3) status—the legal right to operate as a non-profit organization. But the story begins way before... the HavenHouse roots can be traced back to an orphanage that opened its doors nearly a hundred and fifty years ago, as told in chapter one. And what follows is the story of the first twenty-years of HavenHouse, built from personal accounts and the organization's records, and mixed with a bit of legend and lore.

In the book, you will meet the founders and some of the early board members who had a significant impact on the organization; hear stories from the patients and families whom HavenHouse has been honored to serve; read volunteer stories on how they became connected to HavenHouse; learn about the fundraising and friend-raising events that have supported the organization and moved it to the next level; and you will read amusing, soul-searching, and sometimes tragic tales that have made HavenHouse what it is today.

For twenty years, HavenHouse has focused on caring for families so they can care for their hospitalized loved ones. It serves an average of seven thousand guests annually—patients and families—and the guests have come from all fifty states and from more than fifty countries. Its services are available to both children and adults with any medical issue.

And May 2019 was a celebratory month—the 100,000th guest crossed the threshold!

As you will soon see, each chapter in the book is a history within itself; for example, three chapters discuss the buildings in which HavenHouse set up shop since its inception, and another chapter details the evolution of the major fundraiser over the twenty years. And I promise it won't be mind-numbing at all.

I hope you enjoy reading this book as much as I had writing it!

Glenn Sartori

Chapter One
ROOTS

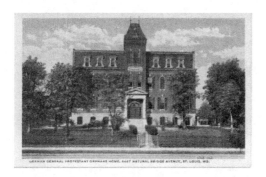

GERMAN GENERAL PROTESTANT ORPHANS HOME, 4447 NATURAL BRIDGE AVENUE, ST. LOUIS, MO.

Finding your roots provides a sense of identity, belonging, and connection to one's cultural, historical, and familial heritage. It's the same with HavenHouse, as its roots can be traced back to a nineteenth-century orphanage in the Northside of the City of St. Louis, Missouri.

In the mid-to-late 1800s, the city experienced the peak of the great German immigration, a cholera epidemic and the pangs of industrialization. Many of those German immigrant families, as other St. Louis families, bore the cruel effect of the events—illness, death and/or abject poverty. The children of many families were saddled with sickness, malnutrition, neglect, abuse, and in some cases, abandonment. A group of German-American men, determined to help the children in their community, founded the German General Protestant Orphans' Association. The mission of the association was to house and feed orphaned children and half-orphans—if the parent of the child or children was a member of the association—and to provide loving care for them with little or no compensation.

On May 2, 1877, the association, a 390-member organization, purchased a three-acre plot of ground in St. Louis North City, on Natural Bridge Road near Newstead, with the goal to build a permanent home for the children. During the construction of the home, the orphans were lodged in a rented house in the neighborhood. Then, a little more than a year later, General Protestant Children's Home, a Dickensian, three-story building at 4447 Natural Bridge Road was completed and opened for business.

The Home always struggled to make ends meet, and their first deficit, which occurred at the end of 1917 pushed the board to seek other income besides members' dues, interest income and residents' fees. The annual picnic, had mostly been a celebratory event, was expanded—the meager admission price was replaced with a charge for dinner, and carnival-style booths were added to raise additional funds. The diamond jubilee picnic in June 1952 was an enormous success and raised the bar for future fundraisers.

In addition to orphans and half-orphans, the Home eventually accepted children of families who were financially distressed, then ultimately, children under the care of the Division of Family Services of Missouri. That evolution occurred over many decades—from the late 1870s through the early 2000s, through a few name changes, and a move from a multi-story building on Natural Bridge Road in the city to a single-story building on Olive Boulevard in St. Louis West County.

The move to the county was a forced relocation. In

1959, the city of St. Louis notified the Home that it was in violation of a law prohibiting the housing of children in a four-story building. The three-story home violated the law because its basement was only halfway underground, thus a four-story building. Most people connected to the Home thought it was nitpicky to enforce that regulation, and rumors flew that someone in the Association had ruffled a city-alderman's feathers.

The city's decree was another obstacle for the organization to overcome.

The board of directors had to find new property, and they did—nineteen acres on Olive Street Road near Mason Road in Creve Coeur. The groundbreaking ceremony, emceed by board president, Walter Kamp, took place on Saturday, May 6, 1961. The building was to be set 250 feet back from Olive Street Road, and was basically one-story with a two-story central administration office section with space for a dining room, kitchen, music room and library. Living quarters for the children were to be in four one-story wings set at angles to the two-story section, providing daylight for each child's room. Then, during the first week in July 1962, thirty-eight children—twenty boys and eighteen girls—moved into their new home at 12685 Olive Boulevard.

Operation of the Home overcame some minor obstacles but no major bumps until in 2003 when the Home faced another challenge—the quantity of children, whom DFS referred to the Home, was dwindling toward zero. Consequently, the board of directors embarked on an urgent course of action: find an alternative mission to care for children and their families. Options considered were—merging or affiliating the Home with other agencies, thereby expanding the client base; using the facility as a home for families whose children were in an extended hospital-stay situation; looking internationally for children and families; or selling the property and becoming a foundation. And as the board struggled with this weighty problem, a reduced staff continued to care for the remaining children at the Home and worked diligently with the families toward a goal of permanent reunification.

After months of soul-searching and meticulous research, the Home's Board of Directors first wanted to make use of the spacious facility and voted to convert the building on Olive Boulevard from a residential childcare facility to a hospital guest house. It was not only a mindful decision—the history of caring for children and their families would continue—but also, a necessary one, as rural hospitals in Missouri and bordering states were experiencing financial difficulties that caused reduced services and even some closures. That meant more families would travel to St. Louis for medical care. It's like the Plato saying, "Our need will be the real creator." Or in other words, "necessity is the mother of invention."

The Home's Board decided to provide the new hospital guest house with a generous amount of seed money to help establish its mission and a lease to the building for an minimal annual fee.

The mission of the new hospital guest house was to provide the comfort of home and a community of support to patients and their families who travel to St. Louis for medical care. Thus, the staff and volunteers of the new guest house would continue the work of the nineteenth-century German immigrants, that is, "hands-on" care and support of children and their families. Whereas, the Home, now doing business as YouthBridge, moved in a different direction. It operated as a foundation and partnered with donors to help charities in the St. Louis region, especially those focused on children.

Three of YouthBridge's board members—Teri Bales, Marybeth Contreras, and Glenn Sartori—and its executive director, Kathy Sindel, volunteered to transfer from the YouthBridge organization to the new entity and support the new mission.

The new hospital guest house named the YouthBridge Family Community was created in mid-2004 and rebranded HavenHouse a year later.

Chapter Two
HOSPITALITY GUEST HOUSES

Yes, this is a history within a history—not that unusual, and as a matter of fact, quite common. Consider it similar to the backstory of a novel's protagonist.

The original idea of hospitality has remained unchanged since the creation of the word itself. Derived from the Latin word *hospes*, meaning both visitor and stranger, hospitality has its roots in ancient history. Hundreds of years ago, when road networks were scarce and traveling was cumbersome, strangers arriving in a foreign land had to rely on either their camping skills or a local person's kindness when looking for shelter. During the age of pilgrimages and the development of major trade routes throughout Europe, it was mostly inns and taverns that offered primitive rooms to weary travelers—their home away from home, surrounded by strangers and yet made to feel welcome.

The first hospital hospitality guest house in the United States was the Kevin Guest House in Buffalo, New York, and it opened its doors on July 26, 1972.

The Garvey family from Sharon, Pennsylvania, arrived at the nation's first comprehensive cancer center, Buffalo's Roswell Park Memorial Institute, in July 1970. Their thirteen-year old son, Kevin, was to start a new experimental drug treatment for his leukemia. While staying in a hotel, Cyril and Claudia Garvey met other families in similar situations, but less fortunate—most slept in their cars and in hospital waiting rooms and ate vending-machine food. The Garvey family knew what they needed to do.

The Institute was in an old section of Buffalo amid homes in disrepair and with many marked for demolition, but the efforts of the family and the administration at the Institute saved the properties along Ellicott Street. The director of Roswell Park and the director of Social Work led a committee to help the Garvey family with their vision for the first hospital guest house. They purchased the house at 782 Ellicott Street on January 5, 1972—Kevin visited the house but sadly passed away nine days later. Today, the Kevin Guest House is still operational, one of many similar buildings on the grounds of the Buffalo-Niagara Medical Campus, and certainly an inspiration for other hospital guest houses across the country.

The most well-known and ubiquitous hospital guest houses are a huge part of the Ronald McDonald Charities. The first Ronald McDonald House opened on October 15, 1974, in Philadelphia, Pennsylvania.

The prior year, Fred Hill and his wife, Fran, arrived at the Philadelphia Children's Hospital to obtain treatment of their daughter Kim's leukemia. They were so impressed with the service Kim received, they wanted to do something for the hospital. The head of pediatric oncology mentioned that many families had to travel great distances and had no place to stay, so having a house close to the hospital would be an excellent way to give back.

Fred, a retired Philadelphia Eagle football player, asked Jim, the Eagles general manager, to help with his project. Jim knew the regional manager of Ronald McDonald and heard about a campaign to promote the new McDonald's Shamrock Shake. When Fred and Jim approached the company with the proposal that they donate twenty-five cents of each shake sold to help build a guest house, the answer was—what if we give you all of the money? Can we name the building the Ronald McDonald House? And that was it. Today, more than three-hundred and fifty Ronald McDonald Houses have been built worldwide.

As hospital guest houses multiplied across the states, the directors formed local collaborative networks to share their successes and failures. The networks were fractured and loosely organized until 1997, when the National Association of Hospital Hospitality Houses was formed with its clunky acronym NAHHH. The association provides a professional network that includes online and in-person forums and conferences, opportunity for certification, and advocacy when required.

The Kevin Guest House started it all, and in the Saint Louis area, HavenHouse became one of a handful of hospital guest houses—but the only one that serves patients of all ages and all diagnoses. For twenty years, through generous donations and community support, HavenHouse has been able to give families sleeping in hospital waiting rooms, an away-from-home option. It has eliminated the burden of affording food while traveling and alleviated expensive transportation to and from the hospital.

The history of the first twenty years of HavenHouse is told in the following chapters.

Chapter Three
MEET THE FOUNDERS

In order for a non-profit to be licensed, its board of directors must consist of a minimum of three members. Three board members from YouthBridge volunteered to serve on the new board of directors of HavenHouse: Glenn Sartori, Marybeth Contreras and Teri Bales. But there was a glitch—almost immediately after volunteering to be on this new board, Teri Bales was relocated from St. Louis.

Kathy Sindel had a friend named Larry Keith, who had the skills needed to become a member of the HavenHouse board. She asked him, and he enthusiastically volunteered to take Teri's place.

Therefore, the following four people were the founders of HavenHouse:

Glenn Sartori – the first president of the board. Glenn received his BS and MS degrees in electrical engineering from St. Louis University. He had recently retired from a 40-year career with McDonnell Douglas/Boeing, where he served in the electronic design division. He has gone on to write – first college textbooks in engineering and later mystery novels and memoirs. As of the writing of this book, he remains an active member of the board of HavenHouse. He and his wife, Rosanne, live in west St. Louis County.

Marybeth Contreras – the first vice-president/
secretary of the board. During college and beyond,
Marybeth had always been a community-conscious
individual who wanted to give back. As a proud
member of the Junior League of St. Louis, she
engaged in volunteerism and civic affairs. After
serving for one year on the board, she resigned to
move with her husband, Mark, who had taken a
new job in Ohio. She has continued to volunteer at
a variety of organizations in her new location.

Larry Keith – the first treasurer of the board. Larry
received his BS and MS degrees in engineering and
then worked for the Anheuser-Busch Companies as
the Director of Environmental Engineering. After
serving five years on the board, he resigned, and
soon after that, he and his wife, Mary Jo, move to
Florida, where they enjoy the sun and their life-
long passion for biking.

Kathy Sindel – the first executive director. After
a two-year stint at the Division of Family Services,
she returned to college and earned an MSW degree.
She then worked with General Protestant Children's
Home (later known as YouthBridge) for more than
ten years—working first as a social worker and later
as executive director. Kathy left the YouthBridge
organization to become the first executive director
of HavenHouse, where she worked for the next
thirteen years. Since her retirement in 2018, Kathy
and her husband, Charley, who live in Webster
Groves, have had more time to spend with their
family and their enjoyment of sports.

Chapter Four
BRICK-AND-MORTAR
PART 1

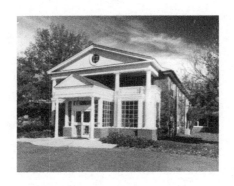

Everyone has a first home.

And nearly everyone remembers where they lived during their growing-up years—their home's layout, where they slept, where they watched TV, and the kitchen, where meals and conversations were shared with family and friends and the place to grab a bite to eat and go. That was the same for the first home of HavenHouse.

The building was atypical from other hospital guest houses, which usually have two or more floors. The building was flat-roofed, basically a single-story structure that sat on a nineteen-acre piece of property on Olive Boulevard in West St. Louis County—the land and building was owned by YouthBridge. And on the same property, behind HavenHouse, was Good Shepherd School for Children—an early childhood education and therapy facility. YouthBridge had envisioned a campus setting for multiple non-profits.

Built in 1962, the home had a circular asphalt driveway, faced Olive Boulevard—a popular east-west thoroughfare—and was separated from the road by a huge lawn, dotted with leafy trees and pines—a picturesque island in the sea of commercial buildings. The guests loved its location—it was in walking distance of a pharmacy, a grocery store, and a fast-food restaurant.

How about a tour?

Stepping into a small foyer, guests were buzzed into the reception area then greeted by a friendly face behind the counter—possibly one of the many HavenHouse volunteers. After signing in, the guests were escorted to their rooms, down a corridor flanked with several staff offices—and into a circular room, a hub of sorts. It provided access to the four wings of bedrooms, aptly named after birds—Cardinal, Bluebird, Robin and Oriole. Each wing has seven guest bedrooms, a small kitchen, a large room with sofas and a TV—a gathering and socializing place for the families—and a common laundry room. Each bedroom had a huge window with a view of the grounds, a private bath, one or two beds, and a closet.

Continuing the tour of the home, a pair of double doors in the hub opened into a lovely dining area. Long tables and square tables dotted the area, along with a buffet-style serving island, and upright coolers that housed cold drinks and food to go. Floor to ceiling windows gave the guests a view of the gardens and the grounds—a welcoming and delightful place to enjoy a meal, a cup of coffee, or just relax.

On the far side of the dining area, a swinging door opened into a large, commercial-style kitchen— Georgia's realm. Georgia McGee had been the cook for the residents of the Children's Home, and transitioned to the food preparer/server for the guests at HavenHouse.

The building housed amenities, not typically found in other hospital guest houses—a full size gymnasium, a computer/library room, a workout room with exercise equipment, and an art room stocked with many essential supplies.

Complimentary shuttle rides were available to and from all of the area hospitals, options for elementary and high school enrollment for long-term-stay families, and connections to counseling centers and faith communities were available.

Since many of the families were from small towns, they loved HavenHouse's location—the serene grounds, twittering birds in the trees, an occasional deer or two, and a scurry of squirrels—a far cry from the concrete jungle of the hospital campuses.

Although the building provided a peaceful environment, it was decades old and maintenance problems would occasionally spring up—some that one would expect, but others required instant attention, like the building's roof.

Being a flat-roofed building, it was prone to leaks. Even though the roof had been repaired and resealed many times, rain water found its way into places it shouldn't be—along ceiling tiles and onto the floor. Buckets were occasionally placed around the building to collect the dripping water. In fact, the drip-drip-drip became part of the ambiance— guests ignored the buckets, smiled as they stepped around them, and the staff regularly emptied them like seamen bailing out a ship taking water.

There was more water drama on a weekend in July 2015—why is it always on a weekend?—HavenHouse was without water, and the weekend staff called in the big gun—Paula. It turned out that a pipe had broken behind the building, but thanks to Burger King, HavenHouse was able to remain open until the county water company made a repair. The fast-food restaurant was a next-door neighbor, and the owner allowed the staff and the guests to use their restrooms. When the water returned, everyone breathed a sigh of relief, but unknown to the staff, that inconvenience was a precursor of big time trouble to come.

That same year, in mid-September, HavenHouse was again without water. Then, when the water again flowed, it came back with a vengeance. Some toilets ran continuously, brown-colored water flowed into sinks and tubs, and water pressure varied throughout the facility. The guests were moved into local hotels, and operations shut down for ten days. It was a disaster—sink holes opened up behind the building and water poured through the ceiling tiles in the common area. Over days, a crew of plumbers worked outside to repair a pipe that had caused the sinkhole, another crew repaired broken toilets and faucets, followed by a herculean effort to clean up the premises before the guests returned.

The staff was overjoyed when October arrived.

Chapter Five
BECOMING HAVENHOUSE

From the moment of HavenHouse's inception, the founders faced two enormous tasks: one, convert the building from dormitory-style rooms into an inviting home for patients and their families; and two, market themselves to the community since they were an unknown entity.

Enter Mattress Giant—HavenHouse's first major in-kind donor.

In the strip mall next to HavenHouse was a Mattress Giant store. The store manager was enthusiastic about the mission and convinced his boss to help, and as it turned out, it became the company's largest donation. On a Saturday morning, in June 2004, a huge Mattress Giant truck, loaded with bed frames, box springs and mattresses, rumbled onto the HavenHouse driveway. Company employees, the HavenHouse founders, and a handful of volunteers brought out the old and carried in the new, converting seven rooms (one wing of the building) into hotel-style bedrooms for patients and their families. It was an exhausting but rewarding effort—drinks and pizza were enjoyed by all for a job well done.

HavenHouse was open for business!

The executive director, Kathy Sindel, focused on her next task—hire staff. The first team consisted of the following: Emily McLean - Business Manager, Julie Gaebe - Development Director, Wanda Robinson - House Manager and her staff—some had previously worked with the children at the Home—and Georgia McGee - Dietary Manager/Cook, or as she preferred "Miss Georgia."

Next, they had to fill the rooms with patients and their families.

The policy was that first-time guests must be referred by a hospital social-worker, but repeat guests could reserve a room through a phone call, email or online. HavenHouse welcomed its first families in the summer of 2004. How did that happen so quickly? Well... Kathy Sindel was well-known and respected in the community for her social-service skills and her unbounded enthusiasm and compassion. So... using her contacts in the community, she convinced local hospital social-workers to consider referring patients and their families to HavenHouse. She also enlisted four MBA students from Washington University to develop a marketing plan, which served as their class project. These students helped the staff and the board to form plans to get HavenHouse known in the community and worked on how to let hospitals, doctors, and families know what was offered. Brochures were produced to communicate what HavenHouse provided and had the following key points, which are in effect today.

• Low-Cost Lodging: Families could be with their loved one through every step of their medical journey without concern for where they'd rest at the end of the day. The HavenHouse mission would serve patients of all socio-economic groups, but especially benefit economically-stressed families, who already lived at poverty levels, had additional financial burdens like hospitals bills and decent meals.

• Free Shuttle Service: This program offered stress-free transportation to and from any hospital in the region. Families would have peace of mind knowing they'd make it to the appointment or to visit loved ones with ease, even in an unknown city.

• Meal Program: Families would never worry about where or when to find the next meal as they juggled appointments and hospital visits.

• On-site Support: Caring staff and dedicated volunteers were available seven days a week to offer helpful support and ease anxiety related to medical issues.

All of these services were offered with a limited staff and much-needed volunteers, plus the staff handled the occasional bump in the road with care and expediency, like the displaced families from Hurricane Katrina. Although the organization had been open for less than a year, it stepped up to help. In light of that natural catastrophe, shelter for hurricane victims was in desperate need. HavenHouse allocated a number of rooms for refugee families who were cosponsored by a school or a hospital. Even though no victims were sheltered in HavenHouse, the community lauded it for its generous gesture.

The staff stepped in whenever a family needed emotional support, which was most of the time. But a roof over their heads and food in their stomachs were essential, especially the home-cooked meals. The entire staff was appreciated and loved by the families, but guess what? One of the most beloved staff member was... you guessed it... the cook, "Miss Georgia." The families loved her big smile and kind words, and delicious comfort food for breakfast and dinner. She always went the extra mile to accommodate the families' needs, and HavenHouse was lucky to have inherited her from the children's home. She knew her way around the building's full-service kitchen with its large freezer, walk-in cooler and buffet-style service island.

But HavenHouse could not exist on food alone. One very important aspect was the computer system used to reserve rooms, and know when families were checking in and checking out. It was an antiquated system, inherited from the children's home, and could no way meet the computing demands of the 21st century. The upkeep and efficiency of the system was left to a very important volunteer. John Morris, a retired IT specialist, who volunteered to help maintain the HavenHouse computer system.

He knew his stuff and was always questioning the staff—"Who added this application? Why would someone change this feature? Who moved this connection?"—which put fear in the hearts of some of the staff. But in the end, John put in countless hours, always came to the rescue when called, somehow kept the system running, and updated it when money was available.

As the staff and volunteers were being put into place, the board sought to expand its membership. By mid-2005, the board had grown to nine members, and all rolled up their sleeves to keep the fledging non-profit running. All of them went above and beyond in their roles, serving in a "just-getting-started" capacity. Four board members created programs and policies that were especially needed and impact HavenHouse to this day.

Scott Goodman—a senior officer of Enterprise Bank. He was key in establishing the investments and checking accounts, helping with grants, and bringing many volunteers into the fold. HavenHouse still banks with Enterprise today.

Joyce Coleman—the head of the social workers at St. Louis Children's Hospital. She promoted HavenHouse at her hospital and to her peers at other local hospitals. She was key in increasing the guest population.

Gayle Young—the head of the social workers at Shriner's Hospital. She enthusiastically shared the services of HavenHouse with her staff, the hospital doctors and their staff. She was key in increasing the guest population and is still an active supporter today.

Ruth Williams—a retired Human Resource director at Boeing. She advised Kathy on all staff issues, led the development of HavenHouse's Personnel Policy Handbook, organized and ran third-party fund-raisers, and actively served on the board for ten years.

During the first year, twenty-eight, first-level bedrooms, and two, apartment-style rooms upstairs were renovated to accommodate patients and their families. The HavenHouse staff peaked at seven full-time employees and ten part-time employees, the board of directors grew to seventeen members, and its reputation grew and blossomed, becoming a premier St. Louis hospital guest house—open twenty-four hours a day, seven days a week.

Chapter Six
PATIENTS AND THEIR FAMILIES

When your loved one is in a hospital far from home, your whole world turns upside down. With no friends or family nearby, even simple tasks—finding a meal or navigating unfamiliar roads—can feel overwhelming. That's where HavenHouse comes in—it helps with those basic needs.

HavenHouse is the one hospital guest house that welcomes all patients, regardless of age and regardless of medical diagnosis. Though that sets it apart from others, the majority of the guests have been families with children needing treatment. In the early years, pediatric patients were about ninety percent of the guests at HavenHouse.

Patients arrive in St. Louis by cars or commercial airlines or flown in by Wings of Hope. Many patients for Shriners Children's Hospital and their families arrive at HavenHouse in white vans driven by Shriner members from neighboring states and small towns in Missouri. The transportation of those gives the Shriners the opportunity to meet the patients they are helping through their organization. Since many of the van drivers had been the same year after year, the staff formed friendships with them and even offered overnight

Glenn Sartori

lodging at HavenHouse. Some took the offer and stayed in an upstairs apartment in the building on Olive.

A small percentage of the families came from other countries, and some had little or no English-speaking skills; thus, volunteers of a different sort were needed—enter the women of Great Shapes.

Great Shapes was a women's exercise facility less than a mile west of the original HavenHouse building. Many HavenHouse volunteers were recruited from that facility, because... besides working out, socializing happened there. The Great Shapes members and their community connections were the basis of the Ambassador Committee of HavenHouse. Doctor's offices provide interpreters to communicate medical information to the families, but HavenHouse wanted hosts who could welcome people with little or no English skills. The committee sought out area residents who were gracious enough to be interpreters for the families during their stay at HavenHouse, Some of the committee members bonded with the families and became more than interpreters—they took them shopping or to visit local tourist sites, and some kept in contact with them over the years even after the families had left St. Louis.

Today, some out-of-country guests speak English, but if not, Google Translator is used—AI has replaced the Ambassador Committee. The app works well, and the families are familiar with its operation. But for long-term stays, sometimes the staff reaches out to the community for interpreters, including international students at St. Louis and Washington Universities.

Throughout the twenty years, HavenHouse has formed partnerships with all of the local hospitals, and the number of patients staying at HavenHouse from each of the hospitals vary from day to day as does the mix of pediatric and adult patients. A snapshot of the distribution near the end of 2024 was: patients were from fourteen different hospitals, and the top five were St. Louis Children's, Shriners, Barnes-Jewish, Siteman Cancer Center, and Missouri Baptist with a patient mix of 60/40—pediatric to adults.

The guests seem to love their time at HavenHouse and have written glowing testimonials about their stay. The notes have been collected, shared with the entire staff and the board members, and some have been posted on the website. Here's a typical example, this one is from a St. Louis Children's Hospital patient's family: *"The positive attitude of the staff and volunteers gave us the strength to manage the four weeks in St. Louis. HavenHouse was a strong support to us. Without you, we could not have managed the most important issue—our son's recovery to a healthy life."*

And one from a Missouri Baptist Hospital patient's family: *"My husband and I were very fortunate to have found HavenHouse. It alleviated the stress of trying to find a place to stay and eat during a difficult time. They were very accommodating and easy to work with. The lodging was excellent, very affordable, and they always made sure the families had something to eat. We would definitely like to stay there again if the need arises and would certainly recommend it to other families. Great experience!"*

Some of the families have agreed to tell their story as a written account in the HavenHouse appeal letters, and others agreed to record their experience with HavenHouse on videos, which have been shared with the attendees at the annual fundraising events and some are posted on the website for all to view. (You should take a look.)

Mixed in with the medical worries that the families experienced, there have been unique stories of their stay at HavenHouse. Some of the most memorable involved families from other countries. Here's a small sampling.

The Ambassador Committee of HavenHouse connected a family from Italy with a local Italian organization that acted as their interpreters, ferried them to many of the St. Louis sights, and communicated with them even after they returned home. While at HavenHouse, one particular Italian family was not a fan of the provided American-style dinners, so they made pasta in the kitchen on their wing. The smell of tomato sauce, garlic and Italian seasonings wafted down the hall and drew other families, with mouths watering, to the pasta-making scene.

One time, a priest from St. Stanislaus Parish in the city graciously agreed to interpret for a family from Poland. After he spoke with the family in their room, he met with the staff in the boardroom. "You should know that the man has a huge wad of bills in his jacket pocket. His village collected the money for his child's surgery... I think it's tens of thousands of dollars. Is there a safe here for that money?" HavenHouse had a small safe but could not be responsible for that amount of money. The staff suggested that he give it to the hospital on his next visit, and he did.

Another heartwarming tale concerns a mother and her three-year old daughter who arrived at HavenHouse from Belize on a frosty December afternoon in 2006 for orthopedic surgery at Shriners Hospital. Dressed in tropical wear, they were not prepared for the cold weather, so volunteers gave them coats and winter clothes until they could go shopping. Although the mother only spoke Spanish, the little girl was very precocious and could speak fluent English. Consequently, the volunteers and staff communicated to the mother through her daughter. The family came to St. Louis yearly over the next seven years for more surgeries. Everyone who met the smiling dimpled child loved her, and in fact, she was the poster child for HavenHouse in 2007. After her final visit, the family returned to Belize, where the little girl continued school, graduated from high school with honors, and enrolled in college.

The St. Louis community always steps up to help someone in need. When a Russian woman was asked to be an interpreter for a Russian family staying at HavenHouse's hotel location, she quickly said yes. On a conference call with a staff member and the family, she was able to resolve the immediate issue—but she wanted to do more. She visited the family at HavenHouse, and even brought them a pot of borscht.

Chapter Seven

THE HUNT FOR FUNDERS

Even with the best intentions, a lack of funding causes many nonprofits to fail.

HavenHouse has survived for twenty years because of a generous community, a "never-give-up" staff and a board of directors who adapted to an ever-changing funding-landscape.

In the beginning, HavenHouse received a sizable amount of seed money from YouthBridge Community Foundation to keep the business afloat for a few years, but the burden to achieve financial sustainability was on the organization. And in those early years, HavenHouse was an unknown, competing against established non-profits for a finite pool of funds, and they did whatever they could to have the name and mission recognized in the community.

Board members and the staff "pounded the pavement" like unknown politicians on the campaign trial, seeking recognition in the community and seeking funding support. The staff, board members and volunteers told the HavenHouse story to whomever would listen—from the pulpit of St. Monica's Church, to cold calls to the businesses in the area, and to friends, families and even people on the street. And early on, HavenHouse joined the Creve Coeur Chamber of Commerce, which increased its exposure and led to donations and a handful of volunteers.

Initially, no fundraising idea was discarded—HavenHouse needed money more than the staff valued their time. After a while, the board realized that outside help was needed with their funding strategy. In 2009, HavenHouse hired the Paradigm Shift Studio to advise the staff on where to direct their energy to receive the biggest bang for the buck. The staff became more discerning, asking the question—is the expense and time required to put on an event worth it? In addition, Colarelli Meyer and Associates was hired to assist in defining short-term goals and long-term strategies.

Today, HavenHouse is a known entity, so name recognition is not as urgent as it was when the operation first started. Grants, the direct-mail appeal letters, and annual galas were the main funding sources that helped keep HavenHouse in a good financial position. Yet, in order to remain financially sustainable, additional funding sources are still needed and still sought out. The hunt for funding has always been integral to its existence, just as it is for most non-profits.

During the twenty years, HavenHouse tried a variety of fundraising events, some major successes, some minor successes, and others only brought in a few dollars but increased the number of people who learned about the mission.

So... in no particular order, here is a smattering of them.

Restaurant connections: This is a tried and true fundraiser, where a non-profit receives a percentage of the restaurant sales on a particular day. For HavenHouse, it was *Raising Cane's, Norwhals, Katie's Pizza, Chipotle, Hacienda* and several others—receiving a few hundred dollars per event, but could be held with a small amount of staff time. One restaurant connection was with *Joey's Seafood Grill*, an eatery on Olive, east of the original HavenHouse building; in fact, staff and board members attended the ribbon cutting ceremony in April 2007. The owner of *Joey's* loved the mission and donated a large percent of his opening day take to HavenHouse. (The restaurant is still there today, under the name of *Gulf Shores*.)

Twelve Bars of Christmas: A pub crawl, put on by a national charity, created a fun, casual way for local charities to involve their supporters. HavenHouse, along with four other non-profits, participated in the inaugural event in December of 2012. Each attendee paid a nominal entrance fee, received a swag bag, voted for their favorite charity, and then headed out on a chilly evening to enjoy some adult beverages. At the end of the evening, a portion of the gate was shared among the top three, vote-getting charities. HavenHouse was in the top three for that year.

GO! St. Louis: The Greater St. Louis Marathon usually held in April, often on a crisp morning. HavenHouse had marathon runners, 3K participants, and senior-mile walkers in the event—not a big money generator, but lots of fun and a memory-maker for the HavenHouse team members.

HavenHouse joined the Schnuck's and the Amazon's Smile Reward Programs. Not a big return, but required little staff time.

Walk for Hope: A third party event at Legacy Park in Cottlesville. On a beautiful Saturday morning, participants strolled on the park trails and partook of glazed donuts and White Castles—what could be better?

The HavenHouse Bourbon Raffles: In the beginning, one hundred tickets were sold for each raffle; some sold out in days. One raffle had three groupings of expensive bourbons—only three winners. Another had one hundred individual bottles—each ticket holder got one bottle that was randomly matched to the person's raffle ticket. The Bourbon Raffle continues to be a successful fundraising event.

In addition to monetary funding, in-kind donations are vital to the HavenHouse mission.

In-kind gifts provide essential goods and services without the requirement of tapping into financial resources. Today, the HavenHouse website has a wish-list of everyday personal items for the families and supplies and services for the home—in order to continually have a comfortable and supportive environment.

Chapter Eight
BOARD OF DIRECTORS

HavenHouse board members are volunteers, and a seat on the board is an honor and requires a sizable financial commitment.

Definition: The Board of Directors are the fiduciaries who steer the organization towards a sustainable future by adopting sound, ethical, and legal governance and financial management policies, as well as by making sure the nonprofit has adequate resources to advance its mission.

In the early years, HavenHouse searched for board member candidates, through existing members, friends and volunteers. In 2007, HavenHouse signed up with Board Link—an online organization that paired business folks to non-profits based on mutual interests. Candidates from Board Link were interviewed and many were accepted to board positions, which resulted in an excellent source of interested community people. Over the years, the HavenHouse Board has been fortunate to have many ultra-dedicated members who aren't afraid to dig in and give more time than expected.

Another important responsibility for the board is working with the executive director. The board is responsible for hiring and supervising the director, setting the director's compensation, and holding annual reviews.

The HavenHouse Board initially met monthly—in conference rooms at a variety of locations and via Zoom during the pandemic. Presently, face-to-face meetings are held every other month. A caring and conscientious board has worked to bring HavenHouse from an unknown entity to a premier hospital guest house. The board has always worked together to promote the mission, and fortunately, has been free of detrimental cliques. During the first twenty years, seventy individuals have served on the board, with an annual membership that varied from nine to fourteen, peaking at seventeen members in 2007.

The First Board of Directors

That first board consisted of the charter members—Marybeth Contreras, Larry Keith, and Glenn Sartori—and the following six individuals.

Tom Babington, an attorney. He served as board secretary and had a longstanding association with the staff and board members who had created HavenHouse. Tom was a member of the Missouri and Metropolitan St. Louis Bar Associations.

Joyce Coleman, a licensed clinical social worker. Joyce was the Manager of Social Work at St. Louis Children's Hospital. She also was a member of the American Association for Marriage and Family

Therapy and the Society for Social Work Leadership in Health Care.

Scott Goodman, banker. He headed the financial committee. Scott was the President of Enterprise Bank & Trust, Clayton. He was on the Banking Committee of BMA Missouri Chapter and the American Institute of Bankers.

Hilary Hartung, community volunteer. Hilary was the past president of the Junior League of St. Louis and worked part time for the Service Bureau.

Tracy McFadden, vice president at American Express. Tracy was a member of the American Institute of Certified Public Accountants, Illinois CPA Society and Missouri Society of CPAs. In the community, Tracy was a member of the Junior League of St. Louis, the St. Louis Ambassador's Club, and was a Corporate Achiever for the National Multiple Sclerosis Society.

Ruth Williams, retired business partner of the Senior VP of Air Force Programs at The Boeing Company. Before joining the HavenHouse board, she had volunteered for a variety of other non-profits.

The Board of Directors
at the twenty-year milestone

Brad Burns, President, joined the board in February of 2020. He earned his bachelor degree from of the University of Missouri-Columbia and his masters from Saint Louis University. He currently owns and operates multiple companies and owns commercial real estate in the Saint Louis area.

Ashley Nelson, Vice President, has a bachelor's degree from Missouri State University, a master's degree from Lindenwood University, and received her certificate in Executive Compensation from the University of Pennsylvania. As the Chief Human Resources Officer at American Industrial Transport, she supports domestic and global business initiatives.

Kevin Moore, Treasurer, joined the board in 2024, and had been a member of the Young Professional Board since 2019. He graduated from the University of Dayton with a BS degree in Finance. Kevin holds the position of Vice-President at Asset Consulting Group.

Brian Sabin, Secretary, joined the board in 2018. He earned a BS degree in Industrial Management from Purdue University and a JD from St. Louis University School of Law. Brian is a shareholder at the law firm of Capes Sokol.

Tom Hicks joined the board in July 2016. He graduated from Illinois State University majoring in Business Information Systems and Finance. He is currently at Edward Jones, a director in their technology division responsible for Mutual Funds, Insurance, and Fee-Based processing.

Chris Ching joined the board in 2014. He earned his Bachelor of Design degree from Clemson

University and his Master of Architecture degree from Washington University. Chris is a project architect at Forum Studio.

Virginia McDowell is a graduate of Temple University with a bachelor's degree in communications. She joined the board in January 2010. From July 2007 to April 2016, she served as president and chief operating officer for Isle of Capri Casinos, Inc. She is currently president and chairwoman of Global Gaming Women, a development program to mentor emerging female gaming leaders.

Glenn Sartori has been on the board since its inception in 2004. He has BS and MS degrees from St. Louis University in Electrical Engineering. He retired from McDonnell Douglas/Boeing after forty years with the company and is a published author, having written college textbooks, mystery novels, and memoirs.

Ron Hofmeister joined the board in 2013. He had been the Executive Vice President of Medicine Shoppe International, responsible for global operations of over a thousand pharmacies in the U.S. and ten other countries, until his retirement in 2002.

Jeff Bone is a CPA. He holds a Bachelor's Degree in Accounting from Louisiana State University. He is also a board member on the Investment Committee for his church and is active in the Missouri Society of CPAs in St. Louis.

Zach Warner, holds a Bachelor's Degree in Business Administration from Christian Brothers University in Memphis. He is a commercial insurance broker for employee benefits at Assured Partners.

Katie Goldberg holds a BS degree in Civil Engineering from Iowa State University and an MBA from the University of Iowa. She serves as a Project Executive and Principal at IMEG, a nationally-ranked Building Engineering Consulting firm.

Anne Feeney is the Assistant Vice President of Global Sales for Enterprise Mobility. She has recently celebrated her thirtieth anniversary with the company.

Andrew Genetti, President of the Young Professionals Board, joined that board in 2023. He graduated from University of Missouri—Columbia and currently works in sales as a Channel Account Manager.

Young Professionals Board

In 2008, Jennifer Breckenridge, Director of Development, set out to bring young people into the fold. (Young in this case, means people in their twenties and thirties.) She enlisted her future husband, Derrick Fishering, and the executive director's son, Josh Sindel, to use their networks to reach out to their friends, offering opportunities for them to get involved. Involvement would include— expanding their network and organizing and running fundraisers to support HavenHouse. Thus, the Young Professional Board (YPB) was born.

The board was a group of emerging leaders who were dedicated to the HavenHouse mission and passionate about giving back to the community. Its members collectively fundraise while increasing awareness of HavenHouse's mission and serving as HavenHouse ambassadors in the St. Louis community. Through planning, directing, and hosting fundraising events and volunteer activities, YPB offers many networking and socializing opportunities for its members while contributing to HavenHouse's objectives. Each member helps facilitate the execution of the YPB events and attends all of its activities, and the members have the opportunity to attend or volunteer at HavenHouse's annual fundraiser—HopeFest.

YPB has held a variety of events with varying success. The first sponsored event was a pub crawl, which was a fun time for all. But their flagship event was a trivia night, which has morphed into a Rock n Roll Bingo night, usually held in November. With sponsorships and ticket sales, these events have been very successful. The number of YPB members varied over the years, and since 2011, the YPB president has had a seat on the HavenHouse Board.

Chapter Nine
THE STAFF AND VOLUNTEERS

The driving force of any non-profit is the executive directive.

Kathy Sindel led the team from the birth of HavenHouse, through its growing pains, to an admired guest house for the local hospitals, until she passed the torch in 2018 to Paula Lowery, who was the former House Manager. Kathy and Paula have steered the ship successfully through challenging times, as well as prosperous times. HavenHouse has been fortunate to have two excellent executive directors with the skill and caring attitude that moved the mission forward.

Besides the executive director, the development directors have had a huge impact on the financial health of HavenHouse. In the non-profit arena, turnover is huge for development directors—the average length of stay is eighteen months. In the first twenty years, HavenHouse has had nine development directors—some making a lasting mark on the organization. The first development director was Julie Gaebe, who was tasked to obtain funds for a new non-profit. She worked tirelessly to make HavenHouse known in the community. At the twentieth anniversary, Brooke Noecker leads the development office with energy and innovative ideas, such as the Key to Comfort—a giving program where donors commit to an easy, affordable, automatic gift each month.

At HavenHouse, the Program Director is another key leadership position—responsible for guest reservations and guest comfortability during their stay. Amy Willis fills that position in the twentieth year, and has been a dedicated and compassionate member of the staff for sixteen years.

Today, Paula Lowery, Brooke Noecker and Amy Willis make up the three-person executive team and provide leadership to the expanded staff that covers the 24-7 operation of the new home. Each staff person makes a heartwarming impact on families facing medical crises, and all of them have a passion to support the HavenHouse mission.

Every guest the staff serves is a reminder of why the mission matters. From lodging and meals to transportation and emotional support, the staff is there to make the guests' journey a little easier.

A devoted and enthusiastic staff is definitely needed, but without volunteers, a non-profit would probably not survive. Over twenty years, hundreds of volunteers have given countless hours of their time to move the mission forward. But many of the volunteers donated more than just time—they gave kindness and warmth to the patients and families who rely on HavenHouse as they battle through their medical journeys. Volunteer positions include, receptionists, shuttle drivers, board members, committee members, special event workers, meal suppliers/preparers, and organizers of the wish-list drive for in-kind donations.

What drew those people to HavenHouse? What is their story?

All of the volunteer stories would fill volumes, but for this history book, there is limited space. So, the following people represent all of the wonderful HavenHouse volunteers dedicated to making the first twenty years of HavenHouse meaningful.

Wendy Alexander

As soon as I heard about the mission of HavenHouse, it resonated with me. Having been through serious illnesses with my parents and in-laws, I know the toll that it takes on the entire family. Having to travel and find accommodations for medical treatment can only add to that stress. Providing a safe, welcoming place to stay with meals is such a nurturing act of kindness for the guests at a time when they need it most. I am so excited about the new HavenHouse home! Currently, I am working with the staff on the wish list for the new house.

Jean Book

After I retired from the Special School District in 2005, I was looking for a place to volunteer. I met Rosanne Sartori while I was exercising at Great Shapes on Olive. She exercised there also, and

I think she had some flyers about HavenHouse needing volunteers. She said it was a great place, and they have a wonderful mission. The following week, I went to sign up to volunteer. I loved it there and have been volunteering ever since, most recently at the 2024 HopeFest.

Jeanne Cody

My relationship with HavenHouse began in 2011 when, as a summer service project, our daughter was the first to renovate a room at the Olive Boulevard location. She collected donations, refinished furniture and painted, inspiring other groups to follow her lead. She also worked with Miss Georgia in the kitchen, and when she left for college I took her shift. I helped until the building closed, while also participating in and volunteering with the GO! St. Louis runs, helping with the galas and joining other activities. We continue to be involved in and support HavenHouse because we believe in Paula and have seen up close, the good that HavenHouse does.

David Evans

My wife and I first volunteered at HavenHouse one Saturday morning in 2009. We were working in one of the corridors when we were approached by a very distraught lady. She said she heard we were from Living Word Church and asked us if we would please come into her room and pray over her husband who had leukemia. We were a little surprised but gladly complied with her wishes.

That experience led me to pray every day for this man and inspired us to continue volunteering at HavenHouse. I soon ended up as the leader of Living Word's HavenHouse mission group which grew to about forty people.

I've always said that deep in the heart of every volunteer is the thought that this could easily be my family who needed help in a strange city.

Tom Hicks

I first heard of HavenHouse while I lived in Arizona in 2010. Our friends and neighbors had an infant daughter that required a very rare surgery, so rare that in fact there were only two surgeons in the US that performed it. They chose the doctor that was based in St. Louis and the hospital social worker referred them to HavenHouse. The surgery and their stay at HavenHouse were a success, and they were so appreciative of the support and accommodations of HavenHouse. Being in their mid-20s and parents of two, the financial impact to travel across the country and have a multi-week stay in a hotel would have been a burden, and I'm grateful that HavenHouse was available as an option for them.

About six months later, I relocated back to St. Louis and learned that my boss and mentor (James Markland) at Edward Jones had just become a board member of HavenHouse. I feel things happen for a reason, and this was a sign that I should get involved. When James and Carol Weschler (another board member) retired, I joined the board. I've seen firsthand the financial impact a medical issue can have on a family, and anything I can do to help lessen that, drives me to further the HavenHouse mission.

Ron Hofmeister

My involvement with HavenHouse actually had a very rocky beginning. A very good friend, Steve Wohlert, asked me to consider joining the board several times, and I ducked and weaved, avoiding a direct answer for well over a year. Then, in 2013, Steve and his wife, Eileen, invited my wife and me to be their guests at the HopeFest Gala. I remember vividly being overwhelmed, truly moved, by the incredible caring and sharing demeanor of the people at the event.

Then I visited the facility, and witnessed firsthand the love and passion of the staff as they helped the families staying there. I was hooked. Over the years, I had been on several health related non-profit boards, but usually much larger national organizations. HavenHouse was different, as it was obvious that the daily constant love and passion for patient excellence allowed it to implement good ideas and actions very quickly. Consequently, everyone could quickly witness and share directly with the families in the success. Instant gratification for the effort expended, which is very unique, quite fulfilling, and incredibly satisfying for a volunteer.

I am so thankful for that "free meal" at HopeFest

2013, and the opportunity to serve and advance the fantastic work of HavenHouse for these many years. May God continue to bless everyone at HavenHouse.

Bettie Hunnius

I was the Registrar/Principal's secretary at Ross Elementary School and knew Kathy Sindel during the General Protestant Home years because some of the children living in the Home attended Ross School. Soon after HavenHouse came into existence, I offered to tutor the son of a family staying there long-term. When I retired, I decided to volunteer at HavenHouse. I worked there once a week, calling people to confirm their upcoming stay. I also called organizations and restaurants confirming their donations of food for weekend dinners. I loved working with everyone there. I moved to the Lake of the Ozarks in 2014 and thus ended my volunteering. Although, I did come back one weekend to participate in Go! St. Louis as a member of the HavenHouse team for the 3K run.

Virginia McDowell

You never think a life altering diagnosis will happen to you or your loved ones, until it does. And your world gets turned upside down.

I was an executive at a company in New Jersey, when I was offered the promotion to a corporate position, but it would require our family to relocate to Saint Louis. After many conversations, we made the decision to leave our support network of family and friends, and a neighborhood we loved and head to Missouri.

As part of the process, we had to establish a new medical network. My routine physical turned out not to be routine—a small lump was found in my throat. Many tests later, I had been diagnosed with thyroid cancer. I was shocked, but I immediately scheduled surgery and began assessing the impact on my family and my job.

My husband was working from home, but needed to be near his computer during working hours. Who would help with the kids; get them to practice, help with meals? Who could drive me to follow-up appointments or pick up prescriptions?

We made what contingency plans we could before I headed to the hospital for my surgery. It went well, except for one complication –the tumor was much larger than they thought, and they stunned my vocal cords when removing it. Although the surgeons got most of it, I was told I would need follow up appointments and additional treatments for a couple of years. I had lost my voice, and they did not know when it would return, if ever.

My world was pretty rocked, but then the most amazing thing happened. The doorbell rang and a neighbor we knew was there with a casserole and some coloring books for my kids. Neighbors we didn't know started calling to help with rides, and cleaning, and helping with our gardens. And I realized what Abraham Lincoln had said about "the better angels of our nature" was very true. It took a couple of years of treatments that had me in bed for weeks at a time, and after about six months, I did get my voice back. I learned that we had the village that it took for our family to recover.

When I first learned about HavenHouse and the organization's mission to provide a warm and welcoming hospital guest house for patients regardless of age and regardless of diagnosis, I immediately volunteered to become part of the family. I was amazed at the passion and dedication of the small but mighty staff, and the plight of many of the patients who stayed with us brought tears to my eyes. The battles they were facing were more serious, and the vast majority lived below the poverty line. I learned over the years that we were truly their lifeline as we helped them along their journey. And they became extended family to us.

During my years of service as a HavenHouse board member, I have learned that it is the smallest gestures to a new friend in need that can be so meaningful, maybe just a simple conversation. HavenHouse is a safe and welcoming place to heal, and to know that in times of great need, that there is a village of friends to help families along their journey.

Jerry Rhode

In 2006, I was invited to join the HopeFest committee and after sitting through numerous meetings, I saw the good that they were doing for the people in the Saint Louis area and region. They showed compassion, kindness and energy. Their actions showed me that this is a group I wanted to be associated with for as long as I could contribute.

Brian Sabin

For a previous medical issue, I contemplated traveling to an out-of-state hospital for my medical care, so I am keenly aware of the all-encompassing burden that traveling for medical care can impose on patients and their families. Everyone has been or will be impacted by medical issues at some point in their life, and travel is often required to receive the best medical care. I am inspired to volunteer for HavenHouse because I know that the community and services offered by HavenHouse make such a positive impact on easing the burden faced by patients and their families who travel to St. Louis for medical care.

Rosanne Sartori

It's hard to remember my life "before" HavenHouse. My husband, Glenn, and I began our journey by volunteering at the children's home that eventually evolved into HavenHouse. We had recently retired and had lots of energy and stamina to pour into a non-profit that would help others. Both of us worked hard to get the new program going. We both served on committees that defined the mission statement and helped brain-stormed names that would communicate that mission. Once HavenHouse was established, we committed ourselves to doing whatever we could to get the new program off the ground.

Glenn became the first president of the board and I helped in any way I could. I saw myself as an "ambassador" for HavenHouse. I talked to as many people as I could and tried to get people I knew to donate time or resources.

I also helped with the families who stayed with us. I have so many memories of people who came to St. Louis for medical treatment and I came to realize how lucky we are to live in a city that has world class doctors and hospitals.

Some of my favorite memories are those when I helped brave people who came to St. Louis from other countries. Imagine knowing that your child or loved one can get medical help if you go to a hospital in the middle of the U.S. but you don't even speak the language. During those years, I picked people up from the airport, arranged for translators if necessary, took people to the zoo or the Arch in between their scary medical procedures.

Glenn and I attended every fund-raiser in those early years and I served on many planning committees and worked to do what I could to make these events successful.

The years have flown by and I have had to step back on many of the physical demands needed to help the families at HavenHouse, but I still think of it as "my" non-profit. I still get excited telling others about our mission and am happy that someone sees the good work we do. I am very excited about the new facility on Park Avenue and am proud that Missouri Artists on Main, a gallery where I show my handmade beaded jewelry, has donated thousands of dollars of art for the walls. I will never stop promoting HavenHouse—a "home" that really makes a difference in the lives of people needing our help.

Gayle (Young) Messina

I first learned of HavenHouse when I was Care Coordination Director at Shriners Hospitals for Children. Kathy Sindel contacted me about our interest in utilizing the new hospital guest house. We very quickly learned what an amazing asset HavenHouse was for our families and children who traveled great distances for medical care at Shriners. I eventually became a board member at HavenHouse and was fortunate to participate in the growth and development of this incredible program. I am still involved and supportive after leaving Shriners and look forward to witnessing the continued growth!

Chapter Ten
BRICK-AND-MORTAR
PART 2

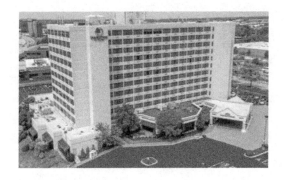

The happy days on Olive Boulevard did not last forever.

The winds of change hit HavenHouse hard in late 2017—the building owner (General Protestant Children's Home, doing business as YouthBridge) informed HavenHouse that most of the nineteen-acre property would be sold, and HavenHouse should vacate the building by the end of 2018, but no later than the end of the first quarter of 2019.

With the imminent loss of their home, HavenHouse embarked on an aggressive capital campaign to build a new facility on the back five acres of the property. YouthBridge had promised to lease the land to HavenHouse and provided a contingent-based donation toward the campaign. The capital campaign committee hired a consultant to help reach its goal and an architect to design the new facility.

Board member, Chris Ching, led the new building project, working with an architect and a construction company to develop design plans and drawings for the new facility and to rezone the land for the new building. The design for the new facility was completed, the land was rezoned, and at a come-

and-see meeting, the neighbors were satisfied with the new building and the HavenHouse mission. But unfortunately, the money didn't follow.

The committee members and the staff had put in countless hours working to obtain campaign pledges and dollars, but the capital campaign did not meet its fundraising goal in the overly-ambitious time-schedule. YouthBridge retracted its lease agreement and their contingent-based donation. The HavenHouse Board decided to pause the capital campaign, hold the collected funds in escrow until the campaign could restart with new focus.

Meanwhile, the building's exit date was fast approaching.

With the capital campaign on hold, the board initiated a search for a partner so that the mission could continue at another location. This effort was led by board member, Ron Hofmeister, and his team of board members and staff. Spreadsheets abounded—possible locations relative to hospital locations, cost versus location, and available space versus locations. All ideas were searched out. Meetings and emails associated with an interim location came fast and furiously. In the end, Hofmeister was the architect of a ground-braking partnership: a collaboration between a hospital guest house—HavenHouse—and a hotel chain—Midas Hospitality The partnership resulted in a one-year contract that allowed HavenHouse to continue its mission at the Staybridge Suites in Westport, less than two miles north of the Olive location. The joint venture was an out-of-the-box idea—reportedly, the first of its kind in the U.S.—and was lauded by the community and other hospital guest houses.

The building on Olive Boulevard was emptied by the end of March 2019, a monumental task, over fifty years of accumulated "stuff." Think of it like thinning out your sock drawer or coat closet and wondering—*where did I get this one? I always liked it. Should I keep it? In the end, you generate three piles— keep, trash, and donate.* The cleaning out of the home was a major effort and accomplished through the tireless dedication of the staff and loads of volunteers. While the building was being emptied, operations were being set up at the Staybridge Suites. HavenHouse was open for business on April 1, 2019!

The HavenHouse-Midas collaboration allowed the continuation of the caring mission at the Suites. The staff and families adapted to the hotel environment and its unique challenges. At the one-year anniversary status meeting with Midas Hospitality, the company delivered the news that the contract would not be renewed. HavenHouse was told that their program no longer fit into the company's goals. Another devastating situation that forced HavenHouse to again relocate, but the board of directors would not give up on the mission.

Stepping up was the Lodging Hospitality Management (LHM) Company. They believed that their organization and HavenHouse would be a perfect fit. LHM signed a two-year contract with

HavenHouse to set up business in their Doubletree Hotel, also in the Westport area. The contract gave HavenHouse a block of guest rooms and two conference rooms—one for the staff office and the other as a private space for families to connect with each other. The staff did yeomen work to continue the mission in cramped quarters. The LHM partner happily supported the mission—attending the annual fundraiser and advertising the partnership in the community. In 2022, the contract was renewed for another two years.

Chapter Eleven
THE GALAS

Just saying the word *gala* makes you smile.

In the non-profit world, a gala is a festive occasion that recognizes the organization's successes for that year, builds a case for continued support, and is an enjoyable event. Attendees donate to the non-profit by purchasing tickets to the event and through activities like silent and oral auctions and appeals made during the evening. As with all non-profits, the annual gala is usually their prime fundraising event. And every year, volunteers, along with the staff, form committees that plan the event, solicit donations and auction gifts, and work tirelessly for many months.

For HavenHouse, the first gala was called *WinterFest*. It was held in the Olive building's gymnasium in early December 2004 and was organized by a small crew of volunteers led by Rosanne Sartori. Local businesses, like professional sport teams, a local television channel, St. Louis Children's Hospital, and families donated and decorated Christmas trees, which were auctioned off at the end of the evening. There were eight live trees, and notables were: a *Very Beary Christmas* tree decorated with small stuffed bears sitting on the branches; two *All*

Sports trees—sport's merchandise filled the limbs; and a *Let's Hear it for Santa* tree—all ornaments were Santa characters. The event was a casual affair, no sit-down dinner, but unlimited amount of finger foods, drinks and lots of fun.

The WinterFest galas were successful but had to be expanded to meet the ever-growing monetary need to provide for the HavenHouse families. So, after the 2007 event, the board decided that they had to up their game and move it to an off-campus location. The annual gala evolved from a casual affair to a sumptuous occasion with a sit-down dinner, raffles, and silent and oral auctions—and rebranded itself as *HopeFest*, a name more relatable to the mission and not tied to a particular season.

The first HopeFest was in January 2009 and was held in the Randall Gallery, a restored building from the Civil War era and one of the more distinct venues in the St. Louis area. Contemporary art was displayed throughout the gallery for viewing and creating conversations during the cocktail hour. However, having the cocktail hour and the silent auction items on one floor and the dinner on another floor proved to be a common complaint of the guests. The size of the gallery limited the numbers of attendees, so a bigger venue was needed.

The next eight HopeFests, 2010 through 2017, were held at hotels in Clayton, Missouri—two at the Crowne Plaza, four at the Ritz-Carlton, and two at the Four Seasons. Each year, event themes became more innovative, like the circus-themed HopeFest, where acrobats and jugglers greeted the arriving guests. At the events, awards were given to the volunteer of the year, a community partner, or to a doctor who had a major impact on the patients and families of HavenHouse.

Some events had live music, local entertainment and a video that introduced the crowd to the mission and to a family who would tell a touching story of their loved one needing medical care and how much HavenHouse meant to them. The videos became a mainstay of all of the galas and many were posted on the HavenHouse website. Also, during those years, the silent auction transitioned from paper biding to smart-phone bidding. It was a steep learning curve for the staff and the attendees alike, and not without glitches, but it was eventually used for the oral auction as well.

Adversity hit the 2018 HopeFest—the first gala at a downtown St. Louis hotel. The event was held at the Four Seasons, a resort-style hotel with a panoramic view of the Mississippi River. But on the same night in the downtown area, there was a Monster Jam event in America's Center and a St. Louis Blues hockey game in the Enterprise Center that caused massive traffic gridlock. Some guests were late for the cocktail hour and the silent auction, while others even missed the salad serving of the sit-down dinner. Then, in an attempt to avoid the traffic for the drive home, some attendees left early, but the Monster Jam was letting out at the same time. And the early exodus meant that less bidders were there for the oral auction.

The 2019 gala was again held downtown at Four Seasons. Why? The hotel understood the unfavorable situation of the previous year and offered a generous reduction in price and relaxed some of their restrictions on what HavenHouse could do. It was scheduled on a night when there were no competing events, but the crowd was relatively small, possibly because of the difficulties previous attendees experienced.

Early in the following year, the pandemic hit St. Louis, and HavenHouse, like other non-profits, hunkered down and put on a virtual gala in 2020 and 2021 with only moderate success—certainly better than no event. Then, in 2022, after much hand-wringing, the HavenHouse Board decided to have an in-person gala —one of the few non-profits that took that uncertain step. HopeFest was held in June at the West Port Sheraton Chalet Hotel. It wasn't a huge money-making success but fared better than the virtual events.

In 2023, the rush by local non-profits to have in-person events left HavenHouse with a meager selection of venues—HopeFest was held at the Hilton at the Ballpark Downtown St. Louis Hotel. The staff and the HopeFest committee were excited about the theme—a Kentucky Derby party with a whiskey tasting side-event and virtual horse-race betting. Most attendees wore derby finery and were having a fun evening until disaster hit. The National Weather Service issued a tornado warning during the silent auction/cocktail hour. People were unsure of what to do, as the wind-driven rain pelted the glass walls that faced the Mississippi River and sounded like hail. The hotel staff announced that the HopeFest attendees must move into an interior conference room, so the guests were herded into a windowless, stuffy room. Everyone was jovial at the beginning of the seclusion, but after being in the room for nearly an hour, grumbling filled the stale air. By time the all-clear signal was given and the guests left the room, the natural flow of the event had been disrupted. Compounding a lack of enthusiasm to get back into the swing of it, many guests left early, thus hampering HavenHouse's ability to raise the funds it had hoped.

HavenHouse abandoned the idea of holding the 2024 HopeFest at any downtown hotel and moved to the Canopy at the Doubletree Hotel in Chesterfield, which provided easy access, plenty of free parking and a more convenient location for many of the attendees. But innovation was needed to get the gala back on a successful track. Two ideas were floated—one, hold it on a Thursday night, which would mean less cost to rent the venue and no conflict with competing weekend events. Second, create a cruise-ship atmosphere with casual attire, making it an easier transition from the workplace, and hopefully introducing a younger group of people to the HavenHouse mission. Because it was a huge success, HopeFest 2025 will be held on April 3, again on Thursday night and at the same venue.

Other fundraisers have been suggested and organized, but the HopeFest gala continues to be the number one annual fundraising event.

Chapter Twelve
JOURNEY FOR JORDAN

In the community of cyclists, there's a popular saying—"Define your life, ride a bike."

People bike for fun—in the streets of an urban city, on the roads in county subdivisions, or on the trails that meander through one state or traverse across many states—or to support a beloved cause or a fundraiser: that was Journey for Jordan.

The Giertz family arrived at HavenHouse on an overcast day in 2011. Their son, Jordan, was to undergo treatments at the Siteman Cancer Center, which were to occur over many months. Jordan loved HavenHouse and its staff and the feeling was mutual. Jordan felt that everyone there treated him like a "normal person," not a patient battling cancer. Sadly, he succumbed to his illness at the age of twenty-two, in his home, surrounded by his family.

"I have this crazy idea..." Michael Giertz said to his wife, Peggy, as he drove back home from church. "... one day, I'd like to ride my bicycle from our house to HavenHouse."

He took his idea farther. In memory of their son, who had been an avid cyclist, his parents, Michael and Peggy Giertz, organized a three-day, 168-mile bike ride that started in their hometown of Gays, Illinois, and ended at HavenHouse on Olive Boulevard. The inaugural biking event, named Journey for Jordan, was held over a weekend in June 2012, and became an annual event and a big fundraiser for HavenHouse.

The money raised for HavenHouse came from participant fees, family and friends of the Giertz's, and moneys collected from people along the biking route who learned about the cause.

The bike ride was meticulously organized with two-overnight stays and pre-planned lunch stops along the way, either at a church hall or a person's house, for well-needed downtimes and home-cooked meals. Days before the bike ride, the Giertz family and their friends loaded up the sag wagon.

A sag wagon is a vehicle that follows a cycling group and provides assistance in case of bike mechanical issues, rider fatigue or injury, or other unforeseen problems that may arise during a ride. The vehicle usually carries a first-aid kit, spare bike parts, food, water, and other supplies to help riders in need. The term *sag* originated from the phrase "sagging along," which describes a vehicle that traveled slowly or lagged behind the others in a convoy. The phrase likely came from the Old West, where a wagon would "sag" or dip down because of its heavy load.

The bike ride kicked off on a Saturday morning from

Gays, Illinois, with a riotous sendoff. It seemed as if the whole town, with a population less than 300, came out to cheer for the riders. The cyclists rode in like-skilled groups, in sort of a buddy system. The first overnight stay was in Vandalia, Illinois—about sixty-plus miles had been covered the first day. The Sunday overnight was in Alton, Illinois—another seventy-plus miles were logged in, leaving less than fifty miles for the final day. The third day's route meandered into Missouri, through St. Charles and onto the circular driveway of HavenHouse, arriving around noon.

At HavenHouse, family and friends of the riders and HavenHouse staff and board members lined the driveway and greeted the arriving bikers with applause, cheers and blasts from party horns. It was a spectacular end to a rigorous, yet fun ride. After group pictures were taken, everyone headed to the HavenHouse dining area, which was set up for a well-deserved lunch of grilled burgers, hotdogs and all of the trimmings. Michael Giertz led the group in prayer, just as he had done at every meal along the way. He concluded by saying that his son, Jordan, had loved HavenHouse and would have been honored to have this event held in his memory. There weren't too many dry eyes of those in attendance.

After lunch, Michael congratulated all the riders and the support team, presented each rider with a certificate of accomplishment, and then shared event highlights to the roars and cheers of the crowd.

One such highlight happened on the second day of the first bike ride: the Sindel family, experienced riders, had pulled out ahead with the idea of speeding up and meeting the group at the next stop. However, they were unfamiliar with the scenery, and... you guessed it, they got lost, and ended up biking miles out of the way.

Over the years, there were some minor mishaps, but one was relatively serious. As the bikers pedaled through Creve Coeur Park, only miles from HavenHouse, one rider hit a guard rail and flipped the bike—the rider required multiple stitches on her chin.

Amazingly, the weather cooperated for all of the planned rides, except one year, when the cyclists had to detour about ten miles out of their way to avoid flooded areas due to heavy rains that had occurred the week before.

The first event had about forty riders participating— Giertz family members, their friends, and Kathy Sindel, executive director, and her family. Over the years, the quantity of riders held rather steady because younger riders replaced some of the original ones.

The last ride occurred in 2018—the final year HavenHouse was in the building on Olive. The next year, HavenHouse set up business in a hotel, which was not conducive to the bike-ride finale, and to date, no plans have been made to restart the Journey for Jordan. But one thing remains—a poster of Jordan Giertz and another of his family hang on a HavenHouse wall for all to see. The Giertz family will never be forgotten.

Chapter Thirteen

FOREST PARK SCRAMBLE

Among the meanings of the word *scramble*, there is one related to golf.

A golf scramble is a tournament format where players work together as a team to play the course. Scrambles are typically played with four-person teams. Each player tees off, then the team chooses the best shot, and all players play their next shot from that location, and so on, for each hole of the course. This format is often used in charity events and fundraisers for a non-profit.

When HavenHouse was still located at the building on Olive Boulevard, weekday meals were provided, but on weekends, volunteers were asked to bring in food and serve the guests. The volunteers were often church groups, individuals, workmates, or families. Some formed a lasting connection with HavenHouse, one such person was a man named Dave Morrissey.

Dave and his family were regular volunteers at HavenHouse—they often provided weekend meals for the guests. In a conversation with executive director, Kathy Sindel, he mentioned that he was part of a group that organized and ran an annual golf scramble.

"Some of my buddies and I put on this golf tournament... once a year, in memory of our friend, Scott Oliphant, and I think HavenHouse would be a worthy recipient of some of the proceeds," Dave had told Kathy over cup of coffee.

Scott Harris Oliphant was a person devoted to his family, a teacher dedicated to his students and an admired individual who inspired everyone who came in contact with him. He lived with honor and grace throughout the course of his short life—but sadly, he succumbed to lung cancer at the age of thirty-six. His family and friends decided to organize a golf scramble—the Scott Harris Oliphant (SHO) Golf Invitational—in his memory, with the proceeds going to families who had a loved-one battling cancer.

"That's sounds great, Dave. What can I do to help?"

"Well, Kathy... if you could come to our meeting next week, that'd be awesome."

That was the start of decades of friendship.

At the meeting, over beers and snacks, the group welcomed Kathy and explained that the golf event had progressed from the first one held in 2004, which had been planned on cocktail napkins at Llewelyn's, to a point where a bit more organization was needed. Kathy jumped in, and with the help of the HavenHouse staff, they registered golfers, streamlined the silent auction process, and provided an overall presence during the day of the event. A portion of the proceeds would go to a selected family and another portion to HavenHouse.

HavenHouse elected Dave Morrissey to the Board in 2008 to have a closer connection to SHO. It was also the first year that HavenHouse participated in the SHO golf event. HavenHouse was a partner and recipient in all of the subsequent golf scrambles, with the last one taking place on May 17, 2024.

During the events, HavenHouse staff and volunteers monitored some of the holes and drove the course in the beer carts—thanking the golfers for participating and offering them a beverage. Upon completion of the course, the golfers returned to the Forest Park Clubhouse for a happy hour, where drinks flowed, snacks were devoured, and exploits of the day were exchanged. After a buffet-style dinner, a SHO board member awarded prizes, such as, closest to the pin, the longest drive, and to the first, second and third place finishers. The day ended with an oral auction and an announcement promoting the next year's scramble.

Notables: One scramble had Jay Randolph, popular St. Louis sportscaster, the emcee of the auction. He coaxed credit cards out of the golfers' wallets and encouraged them to be used in bidding wars. The fifteenth scramble was kicked off with the distinctive sounds of bagpipes to the delight of the golfers. The final golfing event, the twentieth, was the best attended, and the rumor was that many golf carts had to be resurrected from storage to outfit the large crowd.

HavenHouse will be forever grateful for the contributions that the SHO Foundation made to the mission. Scott Harris Oliphant will always be remembered.

Chapter Fourteen
BRICK-AND-MORTAR
PART 3

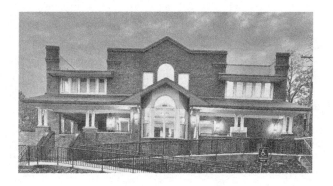

Even though HavenHouse adapted to doing business in its hotel accommodations, the board and staff always considered the hotel environment temporary and was continually on the lookout for its own building. Then it happened—after months of tireless efforts and negotiations.

The hard work of board members, Virginia McDowell and Tom Hicks, and the executive director, Paula Lowery, yielded a collaboration between HavenHouse, St. Louis University, and Ronald McDonald St. Louis Charities. That teamwork resulted in a new home for HavenHouse—a building at 3450 Park Avenue—a former Ronald McDonald House. The HavenHouse Board unanimously approved the contract with St. Louis University. The building and land, owned by the university, would be leased to HavenHouse for a minimal annual fee.

It was a very exciting time and still is!

In August 2024, Paul Lowery received the keys to the building, and the first board meeting was held in the new home on August 22.

The building's unique design has a spacious reception area, staff offices, a board room, small kitchens, a play area, two guest bedrooms, and two 2-bedroom apartments for long-term stays—all on the first floor. There is an elevator to the second floor that has a massive community kitchen, eight guest bedrooms, a play area, a community lounge, and a library/office area. Washers and dryers for the guests, a children's playroom, a lounge area and a large storage areas are located in a finished basement. The building entry is wheelchair accessible, and all of the levels can be accessed by stairs or by elevator. Two huge balconies have outside furniture and a distant view of the St. Louis Gateway Arch—a great spot for grilling or watching holiday fireworks. And outside is great too! There is a kid's area loaded with playground equipment, a peaceful greenspace, and two parking lots—one in the front of the building and a larger one in the back.

Whew! That's some complex.

News of the new HavenHouse building leaked out; it really wasn't a secret, but it wasn't broadcasted because an event had been planned to make the official announcement. Virginia McDowell generously hosted "Nashville Night" on August 27 at Bogey Hills Country Club in St. Charles, MO. The guests—donors, people involved in getting the new home, and friends—were thanked for their support, given the details on the new HavenHouse location, and treated to heavy appetizers and an open bar. All of that was followed by live performances of rock, country and blues by musicians from Nashville. It was a glorious night!

From the moment Paula had the keys in her hand, she and her staff were like whirling dervishes—planning the renovation, rearranging work schedules, and issuing a call for volunteers. It all happened at a furious pace—the plan was to be open for business in mid-December—and volunteerism reached new dizzying heights. The challenging effort of simultaneously running operations in two different places brought back memories of 2019 — the effort of shutting down the Olive building and setting up operations in a hotel.

When Paula put out the call for hands to help renovate the building, Alan, Paula's husband, and Jake, Amy's husband, immediately stepped up, as if they'd been waiting in the wings for this opportunity. Brad Burns, the board president and owner of Wayne Contracting, generously assigned one of his employees to make HavenHouse his job site until his work is completed.

Over the next four months, enthusiastic groups—from businesses, schools and social clubs—and individuals came to HavenHouse to remove wallpaper, paint the seemingly endless number of walls, and clean up every nook and cranny until they were dust and dirt free. It took a village to prepare the house for guests.

The newly painted walls would not be blank for long. Missouri Artists on Main (MAOM), an art gallery in St. Charles, donated over one hundred pieces of wall art—watercolor, oil and mixed media—a huge in-kind donation. Jean McMullen, the gallery owner, spearheaded the donation of the art, and with the help of Rosanne Sartori, the items were collected, catalogued and transported from St. Charles to HavenHouse. The staff was very excited, knowing that the art would be on display for guests to enjoy for years to come, and to let the families know that artists cared enough to donate their art.

In-kind donations for the guest rooms flowed in—pillows, sheets, blankets and quilts, plus shades and blinds as a result of the wish list posted on the HavenHouse website. The list is updated periodically as the needs of the new home and the guests change. HavenHouse has been overwhelmed with gratitude for the incredible donations—the community has continued to respond with abundant generosity.

The outside had a facelift, too! The HavenHouse sign was installed near the rooftop as the St. Louis flag and the HavenHouse flag fluttered in the breeze. The huge sign is highly visible during the day, but when lit at night, it's like a beacon of hope for all of the guests. The greenspace was transformed into a welcoming area with each piece of new garden décor—bird feeders, wind chimes, and lawn art, and new playground turf was installed. The concrete porches and steps were in disrepair as were the handrails. Some concrete areas were patched while other areas needed all of the concrete replaced. And small things, like a welcome mat and a new mail box, were added to give the building a more of a home-like feeling.

While all of the renovation was happening, HavenHouse jubilantly accepted the *Certified Hospital Guest House* certificate. This certification reflects the ongoing commitment to provide exceptional support and comfort to patients, families and caregivers who are served. And to better address the needs of the guests and the house, three committees were formed:

• The Meal Program Committee: This is a crucial committee. Its major task is to recruit volunteers to ensure that the families have two meals a day, every day of the year. That would include on-site meal preparation or readying frozen meals, plus keeping the kitchen pantry stocked.

• The Décor Committee: It was responsible to make sure the house feels like a home. One of their first tasks was to review the MAOM art pieces, plan where they would be displayed, and hang the art after the construction dust had settled.

• The Grand Opening Committee: The grand-opening celebration date is contingent on HavenHouse being open for business, and could be spring-summer 2025.

November 5 was moving day! College Hunks Moving Company trucked most of the office supplies, file cabinets and some IT equipment from the hotel to the new home. It was the first move; the next move was after the last day of operation in the hotel.

Even though the commercial companies that were hired for the repair and renovation had generously reduced their normal service fees (HavenHouse is more than grateful for that.), the effort was still a costly endeavor.

Fortunately, HavenHouse received several anonymous major-gifts that were directed toward the update of the building, including the rehab of the kitchen, reorganization of the existing offices, construction of a board room, and an updated security system. And loads of volunteers put in countless hours of "elbow grease" to make the renovation possible.

Plus a pre-Christmas miracle!

On a Friday afternoon in late November, Paula opened a letter from the Bank of America. She read it twice, and sadly, in this day and age, the word "scam" popped into her mind when money is involved. But in the unexpected letter, it stated that HavenHouse was the beneficiary of a trust, and the dollar amount was huge. If true, it would be the largest donation in HavenHouse history. After much research and many phone calls, the letter was determined to be true. It turned out that a family who had stayed at HavenHouse in 2010, connected with Paula and the staff in a special way, communicating with Paula even after they had returned home. One never knows how kind words and kind deeds affect other people. (I'm sure this could be the basis of a Hallmark Holiday Movie.)

HavenHouse paused taking guest reservations until the Park Avenue home was ready to accept families. The last family left the hotel on December 12, but sadly, the optimistic December opening date had to be pushed into 2025, due to equipment delivery dates not being met. While HavenHouse is extraordinarily fortunate to be in this house, the task to retrofit an old building with no technology infrastructure and a pressing need to bring the building up to code was an undertaking larger than anticipated.

Over the five last months of 2024, the staff and the volunteers have accomplished a lot and plan to keep the "foot on the gas," until the facility is clean, safe and ready to accepts guests.

On January 27,2025, HavenHouse welcomed its first guests into the Park Avenue house.

Chapter Fifteen
THE NEXT TWENTY
AND BEYOND

HavenHouse has done it! The twenty-year anniversary is here. It is quite an accomplishment because according to the National Center on Charitable Statistics reports, over thirty percent of all non-profits close within ten years of operation.

Now, before the final page is turned, the HavenHouse leadership deserves special recognition—it has been an honor to have their guidance and caring attitude throughout the first twenty years.

The Executive Directors:

Kathy Sindel: 2004 – 2018

Paula Lowery: 2018 -

The Board Presidents:

Glenn Sartori: 2004 - 2009

Steve Wohlert: 2009 - 2015

Glenn Sartori: 2015 - 2020

Tom Hicks: 2020 – 2023

Brad Burns: 2023 –

The Young Professional Board Presidents:

Gus Whitelaw: 2008 - 2010

Nathan Keller: 2011 - 2012

Steve Strick: 2013 - 2014

Shannon Weber: 2015 - 2018

Alex Courtney: 2019 - 2021

Allison Benning: 2022 - 2023

Andrew Genetti: 2024 -

As mentioned throughout this book, HavenHouse started as an unknown entity and evolved into a premier hospital guest house—operating in a building on Olive Boulevard for fifteen years, continuing the business in hotel accommodations for five years, then to a building on Park Avenue in midtown St. Louis, within walking distance of SSM Health-Cardinal Glennon Children's Hospital. The staff is beyond excited to have its own home, and they hope that everyone is proud of what has been accomplished to make the 3450 Park Avenue building a haven for families caught in scary medical situations.

HavenHouse is grateful to all who have contributed to the organization over the past twenty years—the financial donations, the in-kind donations, and the countless volunteer hours. Each and every one of you are appreciated, and we hope you continue your support of the HavenHouse mission as we operate out of our Park Avenue home.

The future looks bright for 2025 and beyond.

As patients and their families fill the building, the staff and the board of directors will be working to grow the volunteer base, build new relationships, seek new funding opportunities, and keep the facility spotless and improve it, as needs demand. There will be bumps in the road ahead, but as in the past, HavenHouse will overcome them and continue to move forward.

So... stop by and see the new facility. The staff is more than happy to give you a tour. Or check out the web site, www.havenhousestl.org, for the latest news.

Author's Notes

My path to HavenHouse went through a children's home.

It was a bright sunny Sunday morning in 1992. My wife, Rosanne, and I were driving on Olive Boulevard in St. Louis West County when a large sign, flapping in the breeze, caught our attention— *Sunday Brunch Inside.* We pulled onto the circular driveway and parked in the last open space. The words above the building's double glass-doors read—General Protestant Children's Home.

We were greeted at the door by a friendly face who directed us down the hall and said, "Just follow the smell of bacon." Those words were great directions!

As we walked down the hallway, Rosanne saw a familiar face—Perrin Stifel. He had been a storyteller guest at Rosanne's school quite a few times. After exchanging pleasantries, Perrin explained that he was on the Board of Directors of General Protestant Children's Home, just as his father had been. He invited Rosanne and me to volunteer at the Home.

In the dining area, a mixture of staff and board members stood behind a small buffet-style island and filled our plates with generous portions. We sat down to bacon and eggs, hot biscuits, fruit, dessert and steaming cups of coffee.

After we'd eaten, Kathy Sindel, the executive director, gave us a tour of the facility and handed us some brochures. We were hooked. And little did we know, that morning would be the start of a journey on the evolutionary path of the transformation of the children's home to a hospital guest house. It was one that we have enjoyed every step of the way.

Rosanne was elected to the Home's Board of Directors—the first woman on the board since its inception over 120 years ago. I volunteered to interact with the children—calling bingo on game nights, pitching at their softball games, grilling burgers and dogs for a weekend treat, and teaching financial skills to some of the older residents. When Rosanne retired from the board, I was elected onto it and remained there until I transitioned to the HavenHouse board in 2004 and have been there ever since. It's hard to remember our life without HavenHouse.

Acknowledgments

Thanks to Kathy Sindel, the first executive director. I worked side-by-side with her at HavenHouse for longer than I can remember—her passion, enthusiasm and outstanding organizational skills were tremendous assets during those startup years. For this book, she filled in the gaps in my recollection about the early years at HavenHouse, for which I am grateful.

Thanks to Paula Lowery, the current executive director. She has admirably directed the HavenHouse ship through calm and wild seas. Even though she was totally focused—sometimes barely above water—on bringing the new home on line, she always had time to answer my questions and requests via email, text and a few phone conversations—always following my thank you with, "It's my pleasure."

Thanks to the members of the St. Louis Writer's Guild for their support and encouragement in my writing endeavors.

Thanks to Jennifer Carson for designing the book's cover and for designing and building the interior for the Kindle and paperback versions. She has worked with me on all of my books, from the first one—*Epiphany*, published in 2013 by her company—to this most recent one.

My deepest thanks to my wife, Rosanne, a published author, for her insightful comments and edits to my narratives. Being involved with HavenHouse since its beginning, she contributed much to the stories in this book; in fact, it is a better book because of her.

About the Author

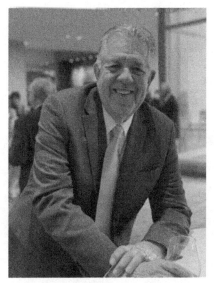

Glenn Sartori retired from his engineering career at Boeing and lives in St. Louis, Missouri, with his wife, Rosanne. After publishing engineering text books, his first novel, *Epiphany*, was published in 2013. *HavenHouse St. Louis – The First Twenty Years* is his second non-fiction book. He has also written his memoir, published as a trilogy plus one.

Scan the QR code below—it takes you to his site: www.glennsartori.com.

Made in the USA
Monee, IL
17 February 2025

12253635R00079